Rapid Weight Loss Techniques

A comprehensive guide for helping you to lose Wight in a fast safe and healthy way

I want to thank you and congratulate you for taking the time to read my book, "Rapid Weight Loss Techniques". This book answers some of the common questions regarding a healthier lifestyle.

Throughout this book you will gain the knowledge for helping you live a healthier lifestyle and potentially helping you to live longer. In these short chapters we will cover everything you need to know regarding: Some of Today's most popular and Successful Weight Loss Techniques that actually work. Thank you again for taking the time to read my book.

Authored by

Richard C.H Yates Sr.

DISCLAIMER AND/OR LEGAL NOTICES

The information presented herein represents the views of the author as of the date of publication.

Because the rate with which conditions change, the author reserve the rights to alter and update their opinions based on the new conditions.

This Book is for informational purposes only and the author does not accept any responsibilities for or any liabilities resulting from the use of this information.

TOC

Weight Loss Techniques

Free Weight Loss programs

The Atkins New Diet Revolution

The Carbohydrate Diet

The DASH Diet.

Eat More, Weigh Less by Dr. Ornish.

The Pitkin Principle.

Volumetric. For low-density calorie eating.

"Losing Weight the Healthy Way"

The key to a healthier way of losing weight is: Do not diet.

"Losing Weight? - Go Herbal"

Herbalife Weight Loss Product: How to Weigh in With Lower Fat

Hypnosis Weight Loss: Some Ways to Stop the Weighting

Dangers of Using Laxatives for Weight Loss

Natural Weight Loss: When you do not have to Go Over

Eat right, keep moving.

The Way to Losing Weight...Naturally

The "Quick Weight Loss Diet" Trend Disadvantage

What Does Not Work

Overnight Weight Loss

Losing Weight Rapidly

What is in a Weight Loss Diet Pill?

Healthy Diet - A Guide to Weight Loss

Drugs that Induce Weight Loss

Weight Loss Exercise

The Advantages of Weight Loss Patch

Weight Loss Plan: The Goal to Go For

What to Know About Weight Loss Products

Samples of weight loss products in the market nowadays

Here are also examples of weight loss products

Program your Weight Loss in as Easy as a Week

The first week

Weight Loss Surgery: Preventing the Health Risks

Surgery at Present

The Concept of Weight Loss Surgery

Factors to Consider

Tablets to Help in Weight Loss

Pointers on Losing Weight Safely

Beware of the Crash Diets

Eat Properly

Pump Up lean Muscle Mass

Engaging in Aerobics

Extra "Push"

On Taking Diet Pills

Why Losing Weight is good

Weight loss prevents high blood pressure, heart
disease and stroke

Weight loss prevents type 2 diabetes

Weight loss helps reduce your risk for cancer

Weight loss reduces sleep apnea

Weight loss reduces the pain of osteoarthritis

What there is to Know about Diet Pills

There are two kinds of diet pills; one is the prescription only diet pills and the over-the-counter diet pills.

Nutrition Notes on Weight Loss Supplements

Weight Loss Techniques

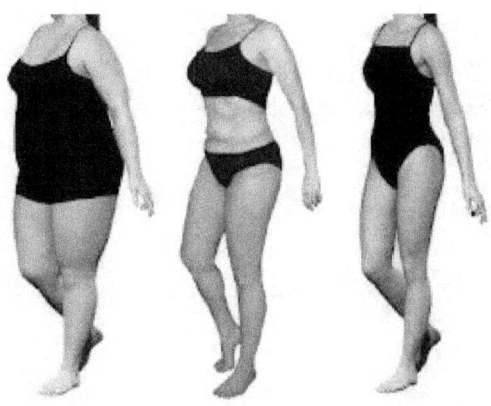

Other than physical appearance weight affects a person in many ways. This could be the overall quality of life, self-esteem, depression, health risks, and physical incapability's.

There are a lot of positive changes once a person experience weight loss. It is for this reason why a lot of people are searching for a weight loss technique that will surely trim down those fats and get a super slim head turner body.

The first thing that an over-weight should do is seek a doctor to recommend the best weight loss regimen.

This will be done after a full physical examination, which leads to the determination of proper weight loss technique.

And to lose weight fast and effectively four aspects of life should be changed: what to eat, how to eat, behavior and activity level.

Here are fast tips that can change an over-weight's life:

First: Fast weight loss composes of a multi-faceted technique that consists of a mindset, exercise, and in other cases, diet supplements.

Begin by learning a diet food plan that can easily be accustomed with. Incorporate an exercise plan that allows even at least fifteen minutes a day like brisk walking, running, swimming, and dancing.

Second: Set realistic approaches. The ability to focus and have proper mindset enables someone on a diet to quickly lose those extra pounds. With discipline and proper mind set, a dieter will never be discouraged and lose focus.

Third: Listen as the body speaks. Each and everyone's body metabolism reacts differently to different fast weight loss programs and plans.

Try substituting one program for another to compensate the body's reaction. Exercise program must be suitable to one's body, as others are not able to exercise as rigorously as others can.

If walking is all that can be done, then walk for this is proven the best exercise. Muscles burn more calories than fats so it's also best to put on a little muscle and looking good too.

Fourth: Eat more fibers for it makes a person full sooner and stays in the tummy longer, slowing down the rate of digestion.

A single serving of whole grain bread moves fat through the digestive system faster. Grains turn into blood sugar that spikes the body's insulin level. Thus, making the body more energized and ready to tell the body when it should stop burning fats or start storing.

Fifth: Keep away from fried foods especially deep-fried as this contains a great amount of fat.

Although fish and chicken appear leaner than beef, this white meat can contain more fat than when a beef is fried.

It is recommended for those on strict diet to opt for grilled food as this does not have or contain less amount of fat after the food is cooked.

Sixth: Takes lots of fluid. Drinking at least six to eight glasses of water a day keeps the body refreshed. Since weight loss depends on how the body eliminates body wastes, the body must stay hydrated.

All in all, discipline and consistency is still the best practice and the key to a rapid weight loss success.

Light dieting, workout, and right amount of supplementation applied in a regular way every day will result in faster weight loss than having a massive action only to be followed a return to old habits as this would only lead to gaining more weight than when the weight loss plan has started.

Free Weight Loss programs

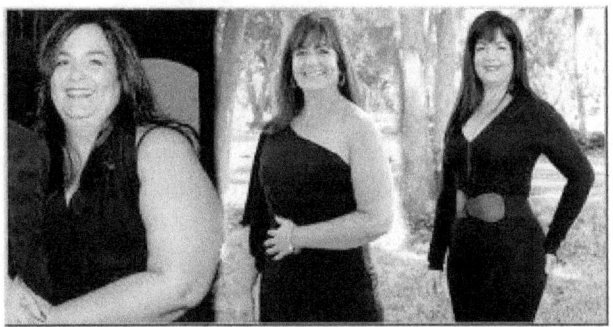

The race to fitness is on and a lot of people are getting into the band wagon. Some people do it to achieve a sexy body, some people just do it because they are embarrassed with the body they have now, while others do it simply to remain fit and healthy.

As such, many fitness programs are out in the internet, in gyms, spas and fitness centers all over. Some are too expensive to afford that one may even lose weight just by trying to work out the money needed to pursue these fitness programs.

One may not have to go to the gym or the spa or any fitness center and spend much just to slim down to obtain that longed for sexy body.

There are many books available in the book store which offers weight loss programs which are convenient and for free, of course the books are not though.

These weight loss programs, or diet plans are gaining immense popularity with so much publicity, testimonials and reviews that one may be confused which exactly to follow.

So before choosing which weight loss plan to follow, try reading these summaries about the most popular diet programs out today.

The Atkins New Diet Revolution

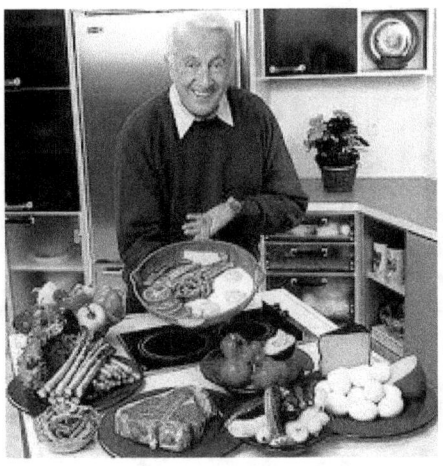

This weight loss program encourages high protein diet and a trim down on the carbs. One can feast on vegetables and meat but should fast on bread and pasta.

One is also not restricted against fat intake so it is okay to pour in the salad dressing and freely spread on the butter.

However, after the diet, one may find himself lacking on fiber and calcium yet high in fat. Intake of grains and fruits are also limited.

The Carbohydrate Diet

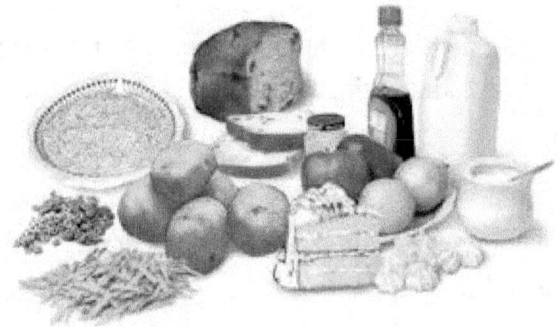

This diet plan advocates low carbohydrate foods. Like meats vegetables fruits dairy and grain products.

However, warns against taking in too much carb. "Reward" meal can be too high on fats and saturated fats.

Choose to Lose by Dr. Goor. Restrains fat intake. One is given a "fat" budget and he is given the liberty on how to spend it.

It does not pressure the individual to watch his carbohydrate intake. Eating meat and poultry as well as low-fat dairy and seafood's is okay.

A go signal is also given on eating vegetables, fruits, cereals, bread and pasta. This weight loss plan is fairly healthy, good amounts of fruits and vegetables as well as saturated fats.

Watch triglyceride levels though; if high, trim down the carbohydrates and tuck in more of the unsaturated fats.

The DASH Diet.

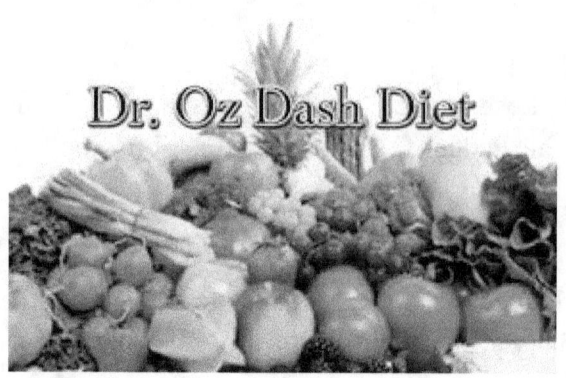

Dr. Oz Dash Diet

Advocates moderate amounts of fat and protein intake and high on carbs.

Primarily designed to lower blood pressure, the diet plan follows the pyramid food guide and encourages high intake of whole wheat grains as well as fruits and vegetables and low-fat dairy.

Some dieters think it advocates too much eating to procure significant weight loss.

Eat More, Weigh Less by Dr. Ornish.

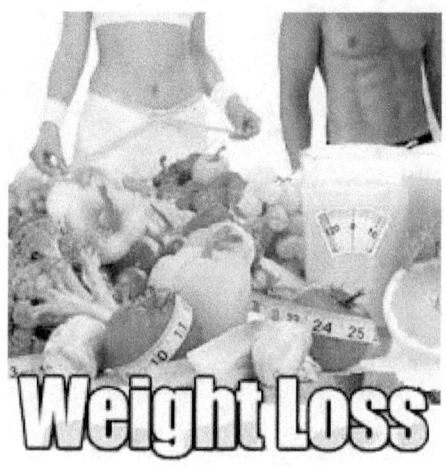

Primarily vegetarian fare and strictly low-fat. Gives the go signal on the "glow" foods but warns to watch it on non-fat dairy and egg whites.

This diet is poor in calcium and restricts consumption of healthy foods like seafood's and lean poultry.

Eat Right for Your Type. Interesting because it is based on the person's blood type.

Recommends plenty of mist for people with the blood type O. Diet plans for some blood types is nutritionally imbalanced and too low in calories. And for the record, there is even no proof that blood type affects dietary needs.

The Pitkin Principle.

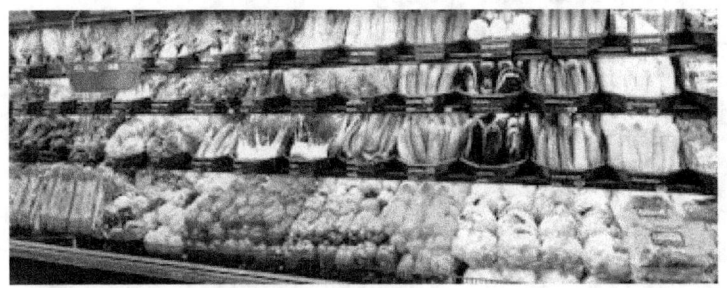

Focused on trimming the calorie density in eating by suggesting watery foods that make one feel full.

Eating vegetables, fruits, oatmeal, pasta, soups, salads and low-fat dairy is okay.

Though limits of protein sources to lean meat seafood and poultry. Although it is healthy by providing low amounts of saturated fats and rich amounts of vegetables and fruits, it is also low on calcium and limits lean protein sources.

Volumetric. For low-density calorie eating.

Recommends the same foodstuff as Pitkin but restricts fatty or dry foods like popcorn, pretzels and crackers.

This plan is reasonably healthy given the high amounts of fruits and vegetables as well as being low in calorie density and saturated fats.

The Zone.

Moderately low on the carbs and moderately high on the proteins. Encourages low-fat protein foods like fish and chicken plus veggies, fruits and grains. It is also healthy but lacking in grains and calcium.

Weight Watchers. High carbohydrates, moderate on fats and proteins. A very healthy diet plan and also very flexible. It allows the dieter to plan his own meal rather than give him a set to follow.

"Losing Weight the Healthy Way"

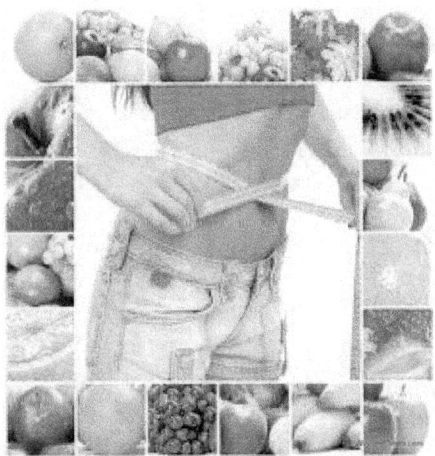

Almost 108 million Americans were overweight or obese in 1999. Until now, obesity continues to be a serious problem and is predicted to reach epidemic levels by the year 2020.

One way to prevent this scenario is to make people aware of the risks of being overweight or obese.

Here are some diseases that you are putting yourself in risk of if you are carrying a lot of extra pounds:

1. Heart disease

2. Stroke

3. Diabetes

4. Cancer

5. Arthritis

6. Hypertension

Losing weight helps to prevent and control these diseases.

The quick weight loss methods which have spread like fire these days do not provide lasting results. More often than not, dieting methods which involve dietary drinks, foods and supplement or pills do not work. If they do, the results are just temporary.

It is better to rely on a healthy weight loss option which will provide lifetime results. You have to set realistic goals and not expect to lose a lot of pounds in a short span of time.

Here are some tips on how you can lose those unwanted pounds the healthy way:

1. Do not starve yourself.

The key to a healthier way of losing weight is: Do not diet.

You may seem happy and feel that you are losing those unwanted flabs on your belly and thighs by skipping meals. But remember that this would not last long. Your body cannot tolerate having insufficient food to fuel the energy that you use up every day.

If you get used to skipping one or two meals a day, your stored calories will be used up instead of the energy that should have been provided by your meals. So if you just eat one huge sandwich in one day, it will end up straight to your problem area (i.e. highs, buttocks, hips).

2. Start your day right.

Mothers always say that breakfast is the most important meal of the day. Have a healthy meal in the morning to jump-start your metabolism.

Your food intake after you wake up will be used to burn fat all day long.

3. Eat small, healthy meals frequently.

Five small-serving snacks per day are better than three hearty meals. Eating more frequently, and in small servings, can prevent over-eating. This will also increase your metabolism and make calories burn faster.

4. Decide on how much weight you want to lose.

Keep your goals realistic. In the long run, it is virtually impossible for you to lose 40 pounds in 2 weeks. Have a mindset that you want to eat healthy to stay healthy for the rest of your life.

Once you have decided on a weight loss plan or program, stick to it and make sure that you follow your own set of dieting rules.

5. Drink lots of water.

Your body needs sufficient water to burn fat and keep your cells hydrated and healthy.

6. Avoid too much sugar.

"Losing Weight? - Go Herbal"

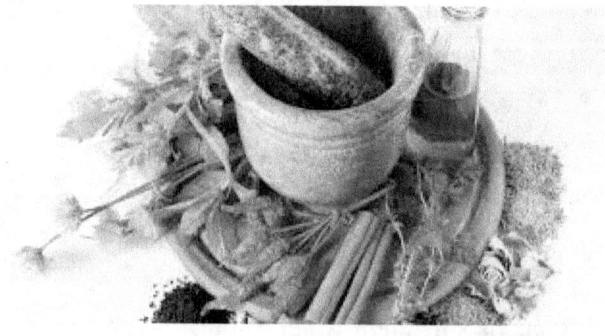

These days, there is a great need for overweight Americans to lose those excess pounds. Being healthy would not only lead them to have a healthier lifestyle but it will also literally lighten their load, and improve their overall well-being.

There is a long list of dieting options available. There are exercises programs, exercise machines, dietary supplements, dietary food and drinks, diet pills - there are even soaps which claim to help you lose pounds while you bathe.

One other available option to shed off those unwanted pounds is to go herbal.

Herbal weight loss products have been in great demand for people who want to lose weight the natural way. However, when you take herbal supplements to lose weight, you would have to wait for a longer time for the results because of the more subtle effects of medicines which came from plants and natural herbs.

Here are some herbal weight lose options that you might want to consider:

1. Herbal weight loss products

There are a lot of herbal weight loss products available in the market now. You can check out the Internet and you will find a lot of herbal weight loss pills and products.

Be careful, however, as there are some products which claim to be safe and natural because they are herbal, but some actually have side effects because of non-extensive research on the effects of these products.

Here are some ingredients and chemicals which make up some herbal weight loss products that you should watch out for, as they might have harmful effects to your health:

Sienna this is an herbal laxative. Sienna is a main ingredient in weight loss teas, and it works by stimulation the colon. The downside effect of this herb is dehydration.

It can also lead to colon problems and can become addictive. Some people, when addicted, are unable to perform bowel movements without it, so watch out.

Chromium picolinate. This is a synthetic compound found in herbal weight loss products.

Chromium is a nutrient which helps regulate blood-sugar level. However, this ingredient, when taken in high doses, may cause damage in the chromosomes. It can also lead to dehydration.

St. John's wart. This supplement increases the production of a chemical in the brain. If not used properly, it may cause eye and skin sensitivity, mild gastrointestinal distress, fatigue and itching.

Although a lot of herbal products claim to be safe and natural, it is better to scrutinize the ingredients and research about the effects of the product itself before going for these herbal dietary pills.

2. Organic food.

In Wichita, Kansas, organic food has found its way to more homes and restaurants. Organic food devotees believe that consuming organic goodies help their bodies as well as the environment.

A person who buys organically raised eggs and vegetables claim to be healthier, and they are not spending money on doctors and prescriptions as these keep them healthier and away from the hospital. This could also be an option for weight watchers, as organic food is known to be kinder to your weight than chemically-processed food products.

3. Green Tea.

Studies show that intake of green tea, or green tea extracts burns extra calories. Also, green tea with caffeine can increase fat burning by up to 40% thereby reducing fat.

This is one good option for those who want to lose weight. In a study done, people who took green tea were found to lose 2 to 3 times more weight than those who did not drink green tea.

These results show that green tea is a natural product for the treatment of obesity. Thus, it also makes for a healthier dietary option, not to mention the good effects that it has on the body as compared to caffeine. A cup of tea gives an immediate energy lift without the side effects of caffeine.

3. Caffeine.

Coffee provides an energy boost to increase fat burning. Caffeine also provides a likelihood to be active, which in turn increases your rate of calorie burn.

4. Immortality Herb

This herb, whose scientific name is Gymnostemna Pentaphyllum, is known to have the following benefits:

> increases healthy blood flow

> reduces artery blocks

> aids healthy blood pressure

> increases the rate of fat burning

5. Apple Cider Vinegar

There are pills and food supplements whose main ingredient is apple cider vinegar. Here are the benefits of taking this herbal option:

> Weight loss

> improved cholesterol level

> improved high blood pressure

> Helps prevent rheumatoid arthritis

Herbalife Weight Loss Product: How to Weigh in With Lower Fat

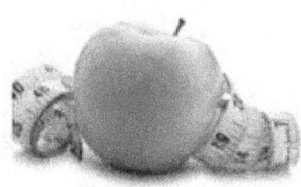 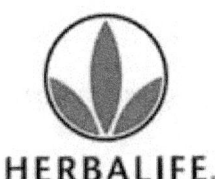 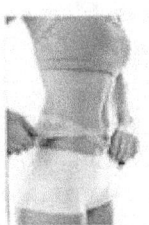

HERBALIFE.

Genetics does play a role in obesity, of course, but not as big a role as you do. Most health experts say that the concept of genes compelling you to be heavy is a myth.

For the vast majority of us, genes may set the lower limits of our weight, but we set the upper limits by our food choices.

Nonetheless, we all know that most of us tend to put on weight as we age. In addition, if there is one thing we cannot prevent, it is the aging process.

But we can prevent eating more and exercising less as we get older. And first of all, you have to have surgeries for food control in your life, strategies that work.

One of the known strategies is to take some weight loss medications. This does not necessarily mean those that are being advertised as diet pills but also those that fall under the category of herbal medicines.

One of the fast-growing herbal medicines especially formulated to help you lose weight is the so-called Herbalife weight loss product.

Herbalife weight loss product is one of the major breakthroughs as far as herbal medication is concerned. Herbalife weight loss products contain the necessary herbs in order to facilitate losing weight.

Some of the well-known Herbalife weight loss products are Herbalife formula 1 strawberry weight control powder, Herbalife diet formula 1 tropical fruit, Herbalife formula 1 vanilla diet slim lose weight, etc.

One of the best things about Herbalife weight loss products is that they are great tasting products, easy-to-use, and is definitely effective in losing weight. Best of all, the prices are relatively affordable when compared to other weight loss products.

To know more of the benefits that Herbalife weight loss products can do for you, here is a list of the advantages.

1. One of the best things about Herbalife weight loss products is that you do not only lose pounds but also inches. This means that Herbalife weight loss products do not just get rid of excess fats but also tone and shape the body built, curbing the imminent re-accumulation of fats.

2. Herbalife weight loss products do not only make you lose weight but also supply you with the nutrients that are needed by the body's cells on a daily basis.

3. Herbalife weight loss products are known to have excellent taste that is why more and more people who have tried it are satisfied with its yummy flavors.

4. Best of all, Herbalife weight loss products lets you eat more of the foods you like without having to worry about accumulating more weight in the end.

5. Herbalife weight loss products are also known to help you lessen the extra calorie ingestion. Hence, losing weight will be more effective.

What's more, Herbalife weight loss products give you the pleasing feeling that curbs your hunger while you lose weight.

The bottom line is that your mission for preventing weight gain, should you decide to accept it, is to eat fewer calories when you are not involved in activities that burn up those calories. Then, try to incorporate these Herbalife weight loss products in your diet.

In the end, you will achieve the ideal weight you have long wanted to obtain.

Hypnosis Weight Loss: Some Ways to Stop the Weighting

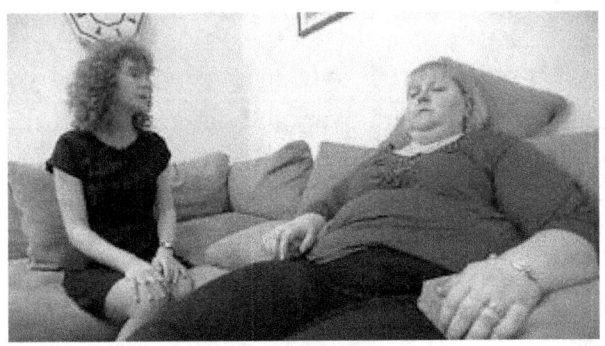

Controlling your weight and avoiding weight gain as you get older are important ways to prevent a host of weight-related health problems.

Indeed, if you are more than 20 pounds over your ideal weight, you are at greater risk for a rogues' gallery of potentially deadly conditions, including diabetes, high blood pressure, coronary heart disease, endometrial cancer, obstructive sleep apnea, and breast cancer.

What's more, most people who are overweight tend to avoid exercise, and that avoidance just adds to the toll paid for extra pounds.

If you have a sedentary lifestyle and are overweight, you are at a higher risk of cardiovascular disease and other health problems. And, if you already have a medical condition such as high cholesterol, being overweight puts you at higher risk for complications.

The good news is that even modest amounts of weight loss can improve your health significantly. Loss of 10% of body weight can reduce blood pressure, high cholesterol, triglyceride, and high blood sugar levels.

Today, there are many procedures that can contribute and help people lose weight effectively. One of the known procedures in losing weight is through hypnosis.

However, many misconceptions have come up with regards to the application of hypnosis in losing eight.

And because it does not involve drugs or any kinds of medications and surgery, many people tend to think that losing weight through hypnosis seems to be one of the safest weight loss programs.

To know more about hypnosis and its effects on losing weight, here is a list of some facts that will give you an insight about what it can do to your body weight.

1. Hypnosis can be an imminently risky if not done properly and not utilize by people who are highly trained with the real concept of hypnosis.

Even if many people tend to think that hypnosis will not pose imminent danger to their health, still, it is important to know that the person who will do the procedure is skilled enough and that he or she knows what factors to consider before doing the procedures.

2. Hypnosis alone cannot eliminate excess fat from the body and, therefore, make somebody lose weight.

Most health experts contend that hypnosis should only be a part of a whole assimilated process. It should never be used as the sole weight loss procedure.

Moreover, one session of hypnosis will only have very minimal results on an individual's weight. When losing weight, hypnosis matched with psychotherapy will be more effective than hypnosis alone.

This is because hypnosis is only a state of deeply relaxing the mind, in which one can still be in control of his or her own body.

3. Hypnosis is one way of getting into the subliminal state of a person. When a person is on the "hypnotic stage," the body is more responsive to suggestibility because of its intensified state of concentration.

However, this does not necessarily mean that through hypnosis, one can already "reprogram" the mind of an individual.

In reality, hypnosis can only run the range from trouble-free relaxation condition to proper initiation managed by a professional hypnotist. Hence, it should not be considered paranormal and magical in its upshots.

Boiled down, people should be more aware that hypnosis is not a sole effective process in losing weight. It is more of a facilitator of various treatment techniques.

Therefore, it should be combined with other weight loss management program to be effective in making people lose excess weight. In this manner, people will be able to lose more weight with a more relaxed and refreshed state of mind.

As they say, a healthy mind is a healthy body.

Dangers of Using Laxatives for Weight Loss

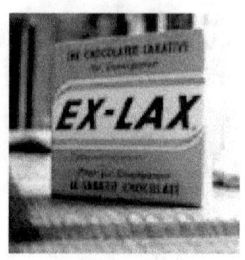

One popular weight loss supplements available in the market today take the form of tea. Stores all over sell slimming tea, dieter's tea and others but all of them are actually the same. They may appear to be effective, but what is not seen may actually harm you.

One of the effects of drinking dieter's tea is frequent bowel movement. This gives people the feeling of body cleansing.

These people may get toxins out of their body but it isn't exactly the only thing that slimming tea actually does to the body. Slimming tea contains herbs which are natural laxatives.

These include aloe, sienna, rhubarb root, cascara, buckthorn and castor oil. These are products which are derived from plants and are used since the ancient times because of their potency in treating constipation and to inducing bowel movement.

Cascara, castor oil and sienna are substances which are recognized as laxatives available over the counter and are also regulated as drugs. Scientific studies show that diarrhea induced by laxatives does not absorb significant amounts of calories taken in the body.

The reason for this is that laxatives do not act on the small intestines where most of the calories are absorbed. Instead, they work on the large intestines.

If taken in large amounts for prolonged periods, it can affect fat absorption of the body.

This may lead to greasy diarrhea and loss of weight. Abuse of laxatives is common practice among people who suffer from bulimia and anorexia nervosa.

While weight loss can be guaranteed by overdosing on laxatives, it may also cause permanent damage to the gastrointestinal tract and the weakening and softening of the bones, a condition known as osteomalacia.

Drinkers of slimming teas may actually patronize the product because they are less expensive and taste better than other laxatives sold in the market. Other people, such as those with eating disorders like bulimia and anorexia nervosa drink dieter's tea because they work fast and produce watery stool and having loose consistency.

Women may even be more susceptible to the effects of slimming teas. Although they may are not known to interfere directly with the woman's menstrual cycle and fertility, they should watch out if drinking them causes them to rapidly shed off weight.

It is also not safe for pregnant women to be taking in laxatives of any kind. Wise and responsible herbalists also discourage the use of sienna and other herbal products with laxative properties for pregnant women and women who are trying to conceive.

One should be wary about these findings because the labeling of slimming teas in the market today can be absolutely misleading. For instance, they commonly refer to the laxative qualities as

"Natural bowel cleansing properties" and not specifically use the word "laxative"

.Some even uses the term "low-calorie" on their labeling. These products in fact, contain essentially no calories or nutrients whatsoever; unless of course, if they are sweetened.

Adverse effects of misusing laxatives in the form of slimming tea generally occur when taken in more than or longer than recommended.

These include nausea, stomach cramps, vomiting, diarrhea, fainting, rectal bleeding, electrolyte disorder and dehydration as well as injury and worse, death.

It was also reported that excess use of stimulant laxatives cause severe constipation and pain for long periods (as much as for decades) due to the colon losing its function. It eventually led to surgery removing the colon altogether.

Natural Weight Loss: When you do not have to Go Over

((Eat right, keep moving.))

You just have read all that you need to know about how to prevent being overweight. That simple set of instructions should be easy to follow, but not for 35% of Americans who are unable to prevent being overweight.

Of course, once we are overweight, we usually want to trim down for a whole lot of reasons, some related to health, others having to do with looks.

In addition, it is never too late to lose weight. But the fact is it is a whole lot easier to prevent putting on pounds than to try losing them later on. And if there is one thing we all know, it is that weight gain is likely to happen if we do not take forward-looking steps to stop it.

Health experts say that most people who are into losing weight usually stray. They tend to go back to their old eating habits even after they learn to enjoy low-fat eating. They tend to return to sedentary ways even though they enjoy exercising.

But despite the momentum toward weight gain, you can stop it from happening, experts say. And there are plenty of good reasons to avoid excess pounds, reasons that go beyond vanity or social acceptance.

In fact, some health experts contend that the significance of excess weight is more than cosmetic. They say that it takes a huge toll on people's physical health.

The Way to Losing Weight...Naturally

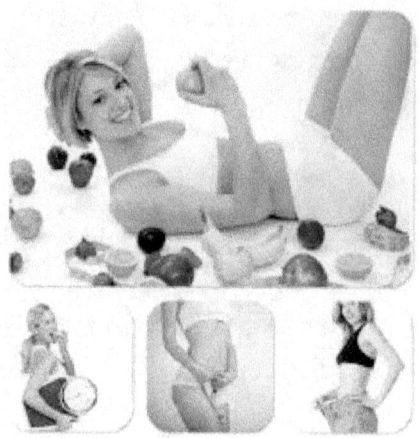

The nuts and bolts of eating right maintaining a healthy weight is not all that complicated. In fact, it is a good bet that most people know pretty well what is best. Hence, losing weight the natural way should not be a problem at all.

Consequently, a reasonable approach for losing weight naturally is to stick to a diet that is high in complex carbohydrates, high in fiber, moderate in protein, and low in fat.

A complex carbohydrate is a baked potato. Fat is the sour cream and butter you should not put on it. Fiber is vegetables. Fat is the oil you should not fry them in. Protein is a lean cut of meat. Fat is the gravy you should not pour over it.

Moreover, health experts say that dietary fat promotes weight gain because it is a very dense source of calories. Also, when you consume excess calories from dietary fat, you store those calories as body fat more efficiently than excess calories from other sources.

On the other hand, it can also help you lose weight naturally if you will not fall into the so-called "fat-free" trap. Manufacturers keep coming out with low-fat or fat-free versions of their best-selling foods, but Americans keep getting fatter anyway.

One of the greatest delusions of the 1990s is that "no fat" means "non-fattening." The truth is you are often getting just as many calories from the no-fat version, even if the calories are not coming from fat.

The term fat-free can be a trap if you start to believe that you can eat any amount of the foods that are advertised that way.

What's more, it is best to respond to hunger with healthful snacks. Health experts say it would be better to try eating every three to four hours, which may mean a nutritious low-fat snack between lunch and dinner.

When you feel the urge for food coming on, snacking on something healthy such as a slice of whole-grain toasted bread is a better alternative. Never skip a meal and eat snacks instead because that is the worst things you can do if you are trying to control you're eating habits and weight.

Remember, if you want to lose weight naturally, you have to keep track of every food you eat and of every activity that you do. When you say natural weight loss means that you do not have to use some accessories or helpful aids just to lose weight.

Losing weight naturally is a process and not a fad. Hence, it would take a lot of dogged determination, self-control, and discipline just to achieve your ideal weight.

The "Quick Weight Loss Diet" Trend Disadvantage

If you wear a size 14 and you blow a bundle on designer size 8 dresses as motivation, you will probably end up feeling guilty, frustrated, and angry if you are not slinking around in it a month later.

In reality, you will do much better setting smaller, achievable targets for yourself. If you must try the new-clothes strategy, go down a size at a time, and do not buy anything you have to take out a second mortgage to pay for.

Because, if you continue to remorse on losing weight fast, you will end up incorporating fad diets or those that offer quick weight loss.

For most people who are not aware of this fact, there are no such things as quick weight loss diets and there is no nippy weight loss for people who want to be slimmer than what their body can provide.

The problem with most people is that they tend to opt for nippy fixes wherein fact these things are not effective at all.

What Does Not Work

Today, there are plenty of weight-loss strategies that are guaranteed to backfire. This is because these nippy fixes instilled on certain diet plans are, in reality, not efficient because it does not employ the right principle and the right attitude in losing weight.

These quick weight loss diet plans are known as fad diets because that is exactly what they are, just a fad. In time, when fashion is over and popularity wanes down, people will realize that the diet they have depended on is not reliable at all.

To know more about these fad diets that are selling like hotcakes in the market today, here is a list of some telltale signs that would tell you not to try it even once.

Here they are:

1. Skipping meals

Does your diet plan require you to skip meals? If it does, then, it is a fad diet.

Abstain from food completely is not a healthy habit. It may even cause some serious complications or problems especially for people who are sick with diabetes.

Skipping meals will only cause a hypoglycemia, or the condition wherein your blood sugar is really low, and will probably only be effective in making you eat twice as much at the next meal.

2. Dieting without exercise, or vice versa

Exercise is crucial to the human body. It is important in the proper blood circulation and other activities of the human body system.

Therefore, diet plans that do not require you to exercise are nuisances. People are born to move.

But then again, exercise alone is not sufficient. Hence, it would be better if diet and exercise will go hand-in-hand.

3. Continuous dawdling

There is no better time to start losing weight. If you want to really lose those excess fats, you have to lose weight now.

Delaying tactics will not get you anywhere and will only make the problem worse. So, if your diet plan suggests a certain timeframe for you start losing weight, chances are, you are following the trend of fad diets.

Boiled down, it is best to rely more on the way you feel than the tale of the tape. This means that if the weighing scale tells you that you are losing weight even if it is slower than you would like, but you are feeling energetic and positive about your weight-loss efforts, then, you are just doing fine.

As mentioned and is worth mentioning all over again, weight loss is not a quick process.

Overnight Weight Loss

The rise in the number of fast foods joints that have a lot of saturated fat in the meals, the use of a lot of refined sugar in sodas and other processed foods and eating food with less fiber have all contributed to the fact that there are more people than before who are classified as either overweight or are obese.

A lot of other factors cause this to happen such as genetics, overeating and as people age; the metabolism slows down making it harder than before to burn the food that was just consumed.

The rate that a person loses weight is commensurate to how it is gained. Rapid weight is not good advisable since it leaves the person with lose skin and the only way to get rid of that would require surgery.

Weight loss depends on the condition of the person which includes weight, health, calorie-intake, age, gender, lifestyle, stress level and routine.

Being overweight does not necessarily make a person unhealthy. It just makes the person a bit unfashionable. Studies have shown that people who are a bit overweight live longer than those who have normal weight.

There is no quick or overnight solution for quick weight loss.

Nutritionists and other health experts will say that a person's weight with proper exercise can actually help lose a certain number of pounds per week the best way to do this is with a low calorie diet and an exercise plan.

The first thing a person needs to do is to choose a diet program designed by a dietitian or another health professional. The patient has to be evaluated before any program can be made. The program usually consists of an eating plan and an exercise program that does not require the use of supplements or one to purchase any expensive fitness equipment.

The best exercise plan should have cardiovascular and weight training exercises. This helps burn calories and increase the muscle to fat ratio that will increase ones metabolism and lose weight.

A good diet should have food from all the food groups.

This is made up by 2 things. The first is carbohydrates. The food that a person consumes should have vitamins, minerals and fiber. A lot of this can come from oats, rice, potatoes and cereals. The best still come from vegetables and fruits since these have phytochemicals, enzymes and micronutrients that are essential for a healthy diet.

The second is fat which can come from mono and poly saturated food sources rather than animal fats. Since fat contains more than double the number of calories in food, this should be taken in small quantities to lose weight.

All diet plans are designed to make the person induce reduced amount of calories into the body. This does not mean that the person has to eat less. It just means that one has to eat smart by choosing the foods that have less calories. This makes it possible for someone to lose weight without the need to eat less.

During the course of the program, the person should still consult with the doctor and other health experts to monitor ones progress. There will be times that it is essential to modify the diet plan to further lose weight.

It is up to the person already to stick to the program to see that it works.

Losing Weight Rapidly

Wanting a slimmer and sexier body is no lofty ambition. Many people have succeeded in sculpting their physiques to make them look healthy and desirable.

However, this end is not attained in just a snap or skipping one night's dinner. For some people though, patience is not a virtue.

They seem not to be able to afford so much attention, time and money to get the body they have always wanted. As a result, these people result to rapid weight loss practices and programs which may not be as effective as these people are led to believe they are.

Fast-track diets are one of these rapid weight loss practices which may not be very inviting as they seem according to research.

Fast-track diet programs, as scientific research shows, are only good while they last. Rapid weight loss often results ironically, to rapid weight gain.

People who undergo low carbohydrate or low calorie diets normally revert back to old eating habits simply because human beings cannot actually live on with this type of diet scheme for the rest of their lives.

Now there is also scientific research showing that rapid weight loss does not imply an individual is losing unwanted excess fat; it is commonly water that is lost with following rapid weight loss practices.

This could cause certain alarm but actually, water lost is regained very quickly. So there is actually zero net weight lost after all.

So one should not be foolish enough to be so gullible with the advertising of certain diet pills out there in the market; especially those which claim to aid lose a whopping amount of fat in a short time.

They will only dehydrate the body. And just so it is clear, the body can only lose two pounds of fat per week, one could be exceptionally lucky if he can lose three, but normally, it's just two.

Another rapid weight loss product out in the market is the slimming soap.

Claiming that these soaps are made from a unique concoction of rare Chinese herbs and seaweed, they assert to help people using them to shed off body fats by emulsifying them upon application while taking a bath.

Some are even specialized like those which promise to give the user "beautiful thighs".

The ingredients may prove to improve the quality of the skin but no research has ever come up yet which aids to prove the efficacy of these ingredients in emulsifying excess body fats.

One more rapid weight loss product out there in the market promises to suppress hunger and at the same time help increase the body's metabolic rate.

It also claims to be able to accelerate the healing process and reduce certain body pains, all these plus its being a very chic fashion accent. Well they are actually called magnetic weight loss earrings.

The secret of this set of earrings is in the magnet, so it says. Wearing them near the ears balances the magnetism in the body therefore one will experience all the above mentioned effects.

Though press releases say that there are actually "studies" to back these assertions up, nothing yet is found in medical journals.

Though buying a set may not kill a person, it's probably not a wise investment. One might as well wear a horse shoe earring for a more exquisite fashion statement.

Bottom line is "no pain, no gain". If one wants a beautiful body, one must sweat it out. And as for those rapid weight loss products coming out on the market, if they are too good to be true, they probably are not.

What is in a Weight Loss Diet Pill?

With all the strenuous activities and sweat-generating regimens that most weight loss programs have, more and more people are enticed to opt for a better alternative, without the trouble of exerting too much effort.

With the advent of diet pills that promote weight loss, people go mad over the appealing advertisements of most manufacturers claim that their product can easily "melt away" those fats and cellulites.

With these pills dominating the market today, who needs to tone those abs and biceps and do some dieting if there is an easier way to lose weight?

With an estimated 60% of the American population that are now considered as obese, these "wonder" drugs are definitely reaping millions of dollars in the United States alone.

Now, the questions are: is there any truth regarding the manufacturers' claims that these diet pills can ultimately promote weight loss? Are they really effective in helping people lose weight? And if that is the case, do these pills also help those people maintain their ideal weight and curb any fat accumulation in the body?

In reality, there are diet pills that can really make a person shed off those extra pounds. These diet pills contain certain substances that were already clinically and scientifically proven to be very effective.

These diet pills are effective in increasing the metabolism of the body, thereby, initiating weight loss. Plus, these diet pills contain certain substances that suppress one's appetite.

However, with so many diet pills saturating the market today, trying to find the best and most effective diet pill can be very tedious. Chances are you may end up choosing the wrong diet pill when your energy to find diet pills wanes down.

Actually, there are only five factors to consider when choosing diet pills that are effective at the same time safe to use. Here is a list of the factors that you need to consider in order to come up with a diet pill that is right and appropriate.

1. The metabolism-boosting ability

In choosing diet pills that will effectively promote weight loss, it is best to look for pills that have the ingredients that will enhance your body's metabolism, or the ability of the body to burn excess fats.

Choose those diet pills that contain alpha lipoic acid, green tea extracts, and "L-Canitine" because these ingredients had been clinically proven to be effective in promoting weight loss through increased metabolic rate.

2. The appetite suppressants

Find diet pills that effectively suppress your appetite. It does not necessarily mean that you will skip meals but you will not just feel hungry every now and then.

This is because obesity usually happens to people who are fond of in-between meals, which actually initiates excessive calorie intake.

3. The calorie stopper

Because obesity is usually due to excess intake of calories in the body, which is more than the recommended amount, it is best to choose diet pills that have the special ingredients that will curb the entry of calories into the body.

These substances are known as "phaseolus vulgaris." This is known to create an enzyme that will efficiently control any excess calories in the body. The enzyme responsible for this wonderful job is known as "alpha-amylase."

4. The metabolic enhancers

It is best to choose diet pills that have the so-called "lipotropic elements" that are effective in eliminating fats from the body. It functions like a sweeper that effectively sweeps excess fats outside the body.

These lipotropic elements are found in vitamin C, chitosan, alpha lipoic acid, and green tea extracts.

5. The water-retention breaker

Effective diet pills are those that contain diuretics. These are elements that avert the retention of water in the body during the weight loss regimen.

All of these factors are, indeed, clinically proven and effective in losing weight. Though, it must be kept in mind that diet pills alone are not sufficient to provide optimum weight loss. Hence, it is still important to do some exercises.

Therefore, with exercise and the right diet pills, you are definitely on your way to a healthier, slimmer you.

"Healthy Diet - A Guide to Weight Loss"

Here are some weight loss diet tips that can be followed anywhere, everyday:

1. Make a delicious low fat mayonnaise by combining one teaspoon of Dijon mustard or satay sauce with a low fat yogurt.

2. Do not skip meals. Skipping meals slicks the body into slowing down the metabolism, attempting to conserve calories during a period where limited fats and fuel are available. Remember that eating increases the metabolism.

3. Stuff vegetables like capsicum and zucchini with flavored fillings or minced chicken, white meat or fish. These are healthy and contain low fat.

4. Take pita bread roll ups or wraps with salad fillings.

5. Eight hours after waking up, our metabolism slows down that is why 30 minutes of exercise before dinner will increase the metabolism for about two to three hours.

This produces an increase in burned fat even hours after the work out is over.

6. Add alfalfa or mung beans to salad to get extra iron.

7. Good cooking and healthy eating begins with learning about nutrition and how to prepare healthy recipes.

8. Learn how to make the family favorite recipes and make sure that fats, salt, and sugar are cut out. Substitute non-fat yogurt for cream, stir-fry without oil and use herbs and spices instead of salt to taste.

9. Consult the doctor before beginning an exercise or weight loss program.

10. Slowly eat and chew each bite during meals as this would decrease one's appetite.

11. Complete three small meals and two snacks everyday instead of one or two huge meals.

12. Use chicken stock when stir-frying. This will cut down on hidden fat.

13. Buy non-toasted muesli instead of the toasted ones. A plate of toasted muesli contains more fat than a plate of bacon and eggs.

14. As much as possible do not remove the skins of fruits and vegetables since most of the nutrients are concentrated under the skin.

15. Warm water with just a squeeze of lemon juice before breakfast get the metabolism going for the day,

this also help preventing constipation and is excellent for the skin.

16. One of the best sources of vegetable protein is from soya beans or tofu. All legumes provide some protein, so include lentils, Lima beans etc. into casseroles and soups.

17. Look for a weight loss "buddy," club, or support mates. This will motivate you to stay and enjoy your weight loss program.

18. Though it's hard at first, try not eating 3 hours or more before bedtime.

19. Make pasta a fast food choice - preparing a pasta meal or salad will only take 10-12 minutes.

20. Chili helps to speed up metabolism - even the milder varieties.

21. Try making omelets without adding the yolks! A dramatic decrease in fat.

22. Substitute baking soda, baking powder, and MSG and soya sauce in cooking.

23. Remove fat by dropping ice cubes into the baking tray. Fat will stick to the ice cubes.

24. Drinking hot water instead of cold water in the morning can increase the speed of your metabolism and burn more calories.

25. Eat before you go food shopping and always prepare a shopping list. Only buy food which relates to your weekly menu plan and don't be tempted to buy goodies.

Make sure that the right discipline is still practiced to promote consistency on the diet plan. This will lead eventually to a healthy life-style and a more fruitful living without the extra fat and extra pounds on the side.

Drugs that Induce Weight Loss

Recent studies have shown that more people are getting overweight every year. This happens not only to adults but even to kids who have just started in school.

A lot of factors cause this to happen such as genetics, overeating, the type of food taken into the body and as people age, the metabolism slows down making it harder than before to burn the food that was just consumed.

There are many ways to solve this problem. Some have decided to undergo surgery, while others have decided to change the dietary intake and exercise.

Since this takes time and most people can't wait to get rid of the extra weight, these people have decided to take the fastest way out which is through the use of weight loss drugs.

In the 1950's until the late 90's, doctors prescribed drugs for weight loss. The drug works by increasing the serotonin levels in the brain that makes the brain believe that the stomach is already full and thus, increases the person's metabolic rate.

It was only after scientists discovered that these drugs had side effects and were related to cause heart valve disease that these were taken off the shelves.

Later on, new drugs were developed and prescribed by doctors and many of which are still waiting for FDA approval.

Most people have known friends or family members who have tried using diet pills and have seen tremendous improvement. The idea that a simple drug can change everything without the need to change the diet or sacrificing anything is very tempting.

This has made consumers spend millions of dollars every year and has given drug companies a lot of money making and selling the drug.

Diet pills can be purchased either over-the-counter or prescribed by a doctor. Even with the advances in medical technology, these drugs can still cause a lot of health related problems which can be unpleasant such as diarrhea and vomiting, harmful such as tightness in the chest and urinary tract problems and fatal such as a heart attack or a stroke.

An overdose of the diet pills can cause tremors, confusion, hallucinations, shallow breathing, renal failure, heart attack and convulsions.

The side effects vary depending on the lifestyle and health of the person and can be minimized as long as one consults the doctor first before buying it.

Should one decide to stop using the drugs, studies have shown that there are also side effects. These include noticeable mood swings, hyper-activity, and pain in the stomach, insomnia and nightmares, severe irritability, extreme fatigue, depression, nausea, vomiting and trembling.

A lot of clinical tests will show that the drugs taken to lose weight really work. But this can only work if it is done with a low calorie diet and an exercise plan.

A good diet should have food from all the food groups. This should have vitamins, minerals and fiber. A lot can come from oats, rice, potatoes and cereals.

The best still come from vegetables and fruits since these have phytochemicals, enzymes and micronutrients that are essential for a healthy diet.

A person can jog every morning or sign up and workout in a gym. Just like taking any medicine, one should first consult the doctor before undergoing any form of exercise.

The best exercise plan should have cardiovascular and weight training exercises. This helps burn calories and increase the muscle to fat ratio that will increase ones metabolism and lose weight.

Weight Loss Exercise

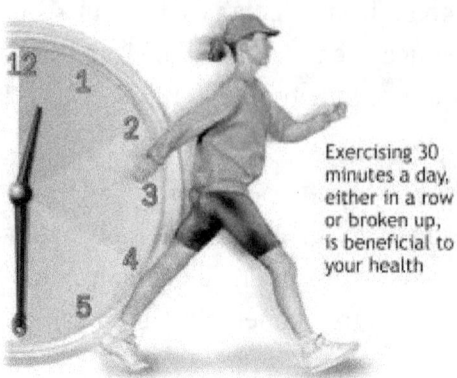

Exercising 30 minutes a day, either in a row or broken up, is beneficial to your health

A lot of us live our lives like penned animals. Built to move, too often we put ourselves in a cage. We have bodies designed for racing across the savannas, but we live a lifestyle designed for migrating from the bed to the breakfast table; to the car seat; to the office chair; to the restaurant booth; to the living room couch and back to the bed.

It was not always this way. Not long ago in the United States, a man who worked on a farm did the equivalent of 15 miles of jogging every day; and his wife did the equivalent of 7 miles of jogging.

Today, our daily obligations of work and home keep us tied to our chairs, and if we want exercise, we have to seek it out.

In fact, health experts insist that obesity problem is probably caused at least as much by lack of physical activity as by eating too much. Hence, it is important that people need to move around.

However, that does not mean that a lap or two around the old high school track will offset a daily dose of donuts. Exercise alone is not very efficient, experts say. They contend that if you just exercise and do not change your diet, you may be able to prevent weight gain or even lose a few pounds for a while.

Nevertheless, it is not something that you are likely to sustain unless exercise is part of an overall program. The more regularly you exercise, the easier it is to maintain your weight. Here is what to do every day to make sure that you get the exercise you need.

1. Get quality Zzzs.

Make sure that you get adequate sleep. Good sleep habits are conducive to exercise, experts point out. If you feel worn out during the day, you are less likely to get much physical activity during the day.

In addition, there is evidence that people who are tired tend to eat more, using food as a substance for the rest they need.

2. Walk the walk.

It is probably the easiest exercise program of all. In fact, it may be all you ever have to do, according to some professional advices of some health experts.

Gradually build up to at least 30 minutes of brisk walking five times a week. Brisk walks themselves have health and psychological benefits that are well worth the while.

3. Walk the treadmill.

When the weather is bad, you might not feel like going outdoors. But if you have a treadmill in the television room, you can catch up on your favorite shows while you are doing your daily good turn for your weight-maintenance plan.

Most of us watch television anyway, and indoor exercise equipment enables anyone to turn a sedentary activity into a healthy walk.

4. Seize the time.

Excuses aside, lack of time is certainly a limiting factor in most lifestyles. That is why health experts suggest a basic guideline for incorporating exercise into your schedule.

Get as much exercise as you can that feels good without letting it interfere with your work or family life. If you need to, remind yourself that you are preventing many health problems when you prevent weight gain; and keeping your health is a gift to your family as well as yourself.

The Advantages of Weight Loss Patch

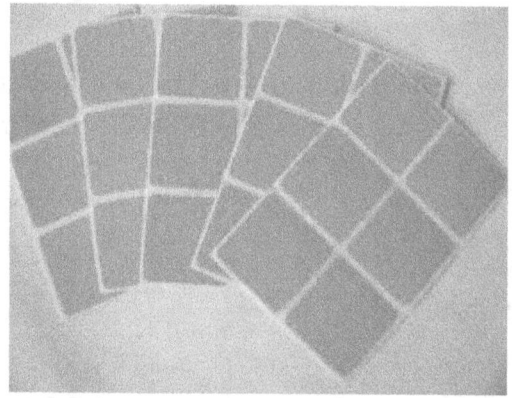

Finally, for severely obese people who have been unable to lose weight using traditional means, the utilization of weight loss patch may be an option.

Basically, weight loss patch is a revolutionary device or product that helps people to lose weight effectively. This weight loss patch, also known as "the diet patch," or the

"Slim Form Patch" are the new and innovative weight loss product that are now readily available in the market.

Its manufacturers contend that the ingredients used in weight loss patches are 100% natural. So, people who will use the product can be assured of a safe and effective weight loss regimen.

To know more about these weight loss patches, here is a list of some facts that can help you understand how it works:

1. It is a biological and straightforward process of losing weight.

This means that these weight loss patches are made from 100% natural ingredients that are why manufacturers claim that these products are safe to use. In addition, it is also simple and easy to utilize.

2. It is not considered as one form of trendy weight loss program.

Because of its viability and clinically proven results, weight loss patches are considered as something that can safely burn calories and fats without having to skip meals or do some crash diets.

Moreover, because it does not advocate people to engage into crash diets, these products have not eradicated certain food groups in one's diet. This means that the person using it is still eating a well-balanced meal.

3. It employs a "cutting edge technology" known as the Patch technology or the Transdermal.

This new technology states that in most cases, the food that enters into the body passes through the different areas inside. In most cases, there are harmful ingredients that were able to enter the body and yet it may pose greater risks.

The point here is that these substances where already broken down into pieces in areas like the liver or stomach, without passing through the bloodstreams. Hence, it poses greater risk to the person concerned.

However, with patch technology, the substances are easily absorbed and penetrated through the skin. It is in this process that the substances are redirected first to the bloodstream, where they are filtered, before they can go to the liver, stomach, and other parts of the body.

In this way, the harmful substances are already eliminated and that everything that passes through the different parts of the body are effectively utilized by the cells, where it is mostly needed.

Moreover, these weight loss patches contain the active ingredients that can effectively help people lose weight at the same time enhancing their health and well-being.

Therefore, for a revolutionary modification to weight loss regimen, it would be better if you will try using these weight loss patches. Buy now and start your life to a healthier you.

Alternatively, these weight loss patches are available in 30-piece package. It should only be worn once a day. Hence, you have a month supply of these products.

Indeed, with the advent of weight loss patches, losing weight will no longer be considered a game for the chosen few.

Hence, with these wonderful, excellent patches, you can now easily lose weight without the trouble of extreme fad diets. Best of all, these weight loss patches are affordable, so there's no reason why you cannot try it out.

Weight Loss Plan: The Goal to Go For

Since excess weight puts you at risk for many health problems, you may need to set some weight loss plans to help avoid those risks and prevent disease.

But what should be your long-term goal? And what short-term goals should you set to help you get there? You have a better chance of attaining your goals if you make sure that the weight loss plans that you will use are sensible and reasonable right at the beginning.

Here are some guidelines from the experts in choosing weight loss plans and goals.

1. be realistic

Most people's long-term weight loss plans are more ambitious than they have to be.

For example, if you weigh 170 pounds and your long-term plan is to weigh 120, even if you have not weighed 120 since you were 16 and now you are 45, which is not a realistic weight loss goal.

Your body mass index or BMI is a good indicator of whether or not you need to shed of pounds. The ideal BMI range, according to the national Institutes of Health, is between 19 and 24.9. If your BMI is between 25 and 29.9, you are considered overweight. Any number above 30 is in the obesity range.

From this point of view, you will need a sensible weight loss plan that will correspond to the required BMI based on your height, because this is the primary factor that will affect your BMI.

2. Set appropriate objectives

Using a weight loss plan just for vanity's sake is psychologically less helpful than losing weight to improve health.

You have made a big step forward if you decide to undergo a weight loss plan that includes exercise and eating right so that you will feel better and have more energy to do something positive in your life.

3. Focus on doing, not losing

Rather than saying that you are going to lose a pound this week, say how much you are going to exercise this week. This would definitely make up of a sensible weight loss plan.

Keep in mind that your weight within a span of a week is not completely in your control, but your behavior is.

4. Build bit by bit

Short-term weight loss plans should not be "pie-in-the-sky." This means that when you have never exercised at all, your best weight loss plan for this week should be based on finding three different one-mile routes that you can walk next week.

5. Keep up the self encouragement

An all-or-nothing attitude only sets you up to fail. Learn to evaluate your efforts fairly and objectively. If you fall short of some goals, just look ahead to next week. You do not need to have a perfect record.

After all, self-encouragement should definitely be a part of your weight loss plans. Otherwise, you will just fail in the end.

6. Use measurable measures

Saying that you are going to be more positive this week or that you are going to really get serious this week is not a goal that you can measure and should not be a part of your weight loss plan.

This is another reason why you should incorporate exercise on your weight loss plan and focus on it. You should be able to count up the minutes of exercise in order to be successful in your plan.

The bottom line is people should make weight loss plans that will only remain as it is, just a plan. They have to put it into action by incorporating goals that will motivate them to succeed.

What to Know About Weight Loss Products

There are a lot of weight loss products that offer that fast weight loss results, however, are these really guaranteed? Could these products live up to their assurance of a fit body?

In US, there is an estimated 50 million people who try to lose weight, unfortunately, only 5 per cent are successful. One thing's for sure, beware of fraudulent claims and extreme high cost because there is no magic to losing weight.

Samples of weight loss products in the market nowadays

·   Diet Patch – this was already removed since 1990's by FDA since they were proven ineffective.

·   Magnetic Diet Pills – allegedly flushes out fat, but not.

·   Guar Gum – causes internal obstruction.

·   Electrical Muscle Stimulators – no proven effect.

·   Eyeglasses that Suppress Appetite – These claims that the projected image on the retina decreases appetite. No proven fact.

·   Weight loss earrings – through acupuncture, suppresses appetite.

There are also examples of weight loss products

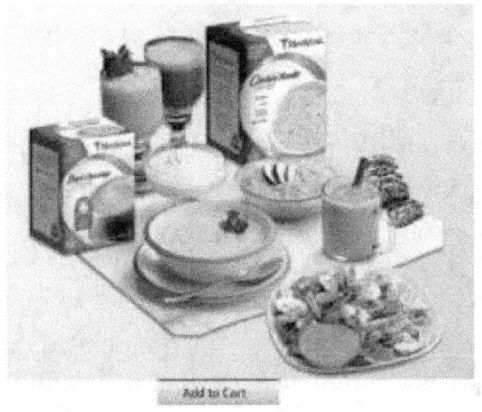

Diet drinks that are mixed with beverages or food are used as meal substitutes. A downside of this is that once a person stopped taking the drinks, they would eventually regain the lost weight after a short period of time due to feeling of emptiness in the stomach.

Another is diet supplements and medicines that also don't work long-term. Over-the-counter pills that compose of phenylpropanolamine hydrochloride may raise blood pressure and palpitation.

Ephedra on the other hand can cause serious side effects such as heart problems, seizure, stroke, and even death. E.g.:

§ Herbalife Nutritional Program – good as two meals, dieters may rely on shakes and follow artificial dieting methods and just don't want food to work into their lives.

§ Mega-Thin 100 Formula – Its formula contains an anti-fat weapon, however, diet is not emphasized that's why it's concluded that it has an appetite suppressant.

§ Nestlé's Sweet Success – recommended taking three times a day and it does not promote healthy eating habits. Weight loss is difficult to maintain once intake is stopped.

§ Ultra Slim Fast – this plan requires regular exercise but does not teach good eating habits.

§   Diet pills with Ephedra and PPA – many of these have enclosed diet plans. Slimming can come from the diet plan and not the pill intake and there are risks of adverse side effects.

§   Chitosan products – contains fibers which were taken from shellfish that may cause diarrhea, bloatedness, and gas. This will only work if a low fat diet is practiced.

§   Chromium Supplements –claim that products will lower blood sugar, body fat and cholesterol but causes anemia and even memory loss. Studies show only minimal or no beneficial effect at all.

§   Green Tea Extract Products – known as strong anti-oxidants that help lower cholesterol and triglycerides, and promote weight loss, however, the caffeine content could cause insomnia and restlessness.

§   Algae Tablets - Spirulina contains significant nutrients that can be an acceptable food when used as part of a varied diet but are very expensive.

§   St. John's Wart Supplement - Claims that it will suppress appetite and promote weight loss but it could lead to gastrointestinal discomfort, tiredness, sleeplessness, and arouse allergic reactions.

§   Glucomannan Products – claim that two capsules before each meal decrease food absorption. Known as food thickeners but not yet proven safe or effective. Weight loss will only happen if good diet plan is followed.

Even if you plan on using over-the-counter weight supplements or even participate in a weight loss activity, the verdict is that you still have to eat fewer calories than you burn to lose weight. When choosing a weight loss product or program, collect as much information as possible.

Program your Weight Loss in as Easy as a Week

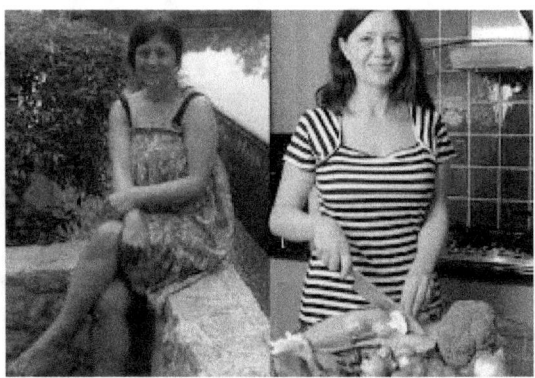

The idea of the program is to be able for you to develop a consistent approach to weight loss as well as a healthy endurance when exercising. The program's objective is to get rid of the excesses in your body, the excess fat. Not the healthy and lean muscle tissues and body fluids.

The program first requires your focus and dedication, so therefore you need to be prepared in both mind and – of course – body. It is highly advised that you first visit your doctor for a check-up before embarking on any weight loss program.

It is important that when starting on any weight loss program, one should be positive enough to work for the results. Some people get impatient easily but long term effects are assured as long as one sticks to the weight loss plan at hand.

Stretch, stretch and stretch some more. Before actually doing those exercises and working out those muscles, a little stretching is needed in order to avoid any injury or soreness in your body.

It is also not advisable for anyone to try too hard. Everything should be done in moderation. Find the level of exercise and training that suits you. It should be enough for you to be comfortable in but not too convenient that it will not be much of a challenge.

The first week

The first day of the program involves a long and steady walk in a little over twenty minutes. After the walk, follow it up with a good stretch. This takes so little of your time for the first day. In less than an hour you have taken that first step to a weight loss program that could work to your advantage.

By the second day, it is good to focus on an upper body workout. This maintains your strength to be able to go through the whole program for the week. On the third day, a brisk walk or jog for ten minutes is in order. For beginners, a lower body workout should be done in the evening.

In the fourth day, a good rest is in order, as well as a good stretch. This lag time should be used wisely though to sort out any negatives in your mindset. The fifth day starts with a good ten minute walk. Exercise the lower body in four sessions of workouts; follow this up with another ten minute walk, and another four sessions of lower body workout.

The sixth day should be spent on a low impact exercise such as swimming. To avoid boredom, do not be afraid to try something new. The last day of the week is a time to solicit the support of the people you care about. Spend time with them or get them to be with you in your long walk. Again, follow up your walk with a light upper body workout.

This is just the beginning though. If by this first week you are able to stick to the program, you have a great chance to further boost your weight loss and stay with the plan until you achieve your desired result.

Try as much as possible to be unlike the people who give up easily just because they could not see the result they want at the time they want – like this moment, today, now!

Patience is a virtue. The same way it took your body time to gain all that weight, think about it as the time your body will have to exert just to get rid of it.

Weight Loss Surgery: Preventing the Health Risks

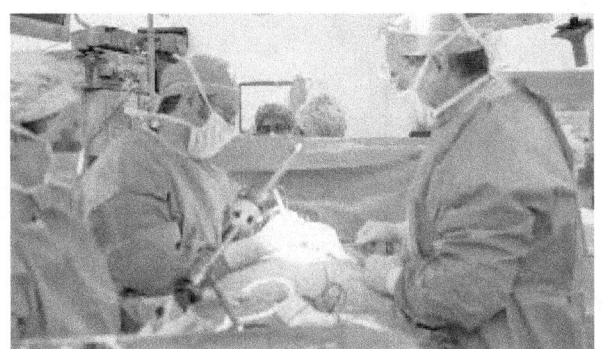

If you have been watching your weight go up and you are worried about the rising pounds, you may be wondering whether weight loss surgery really works. Is it possible to prevent future weight gain by putting yourself on a well-known weight loss surgical operation?

Today, weight loss surgeries are gradually gaining recognition when it comes to losing weight. Many health experts contend that people who are excessively overweight or has slower metabolism would normally require some surgical operations.

Surgery at Present

The greatest progress in the care of the surgical patient has taken place since the beginning of the present century. An increasing knowledge of disease and disorder as a result of research has permitted the development of many diagnostic aids. Some of these depend upon roentgenograms, laboratory procedures such as chemical, bacteriologic, and pathologic determinations, as well as monitoring devices and computer aids.

Hence, the result is that the diagnosis of disease and disorder is made with more exactness and certainty than was possible from the simple clinical examinations of previous days.

That is why people who wish to undergo weight loss surgery should no longer be afraid of the procedure because high clinical standards are now being implemented in every surgical operation.

The Concept of Weight Loss Surgery

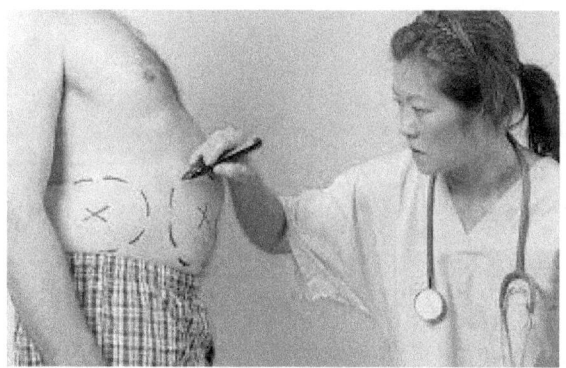

Health experts contend that weight loss surgery is a "major surgery." One of the most common reasons why people would like to lose weight is to enhance their physical attributes. However, it should not be the underlying motivation that they should undergo the process of weight loss surgery.

What people do not know is that weight loss surgery is especially generated to help obese people live longer, healthier, and better.

That is why it is important for an individual to meticulously analyze his or her situation, do some research about the process, and analyze if weight loss surgery is the ultimate choice for his or her physiological condition.

Moreover, it is important to gather further information about weight loss surgery by consulting an experienced and knowledgeable bariatric surgeon or even just an expert family physician who knows the ins and outs of weight loss surgery.

In addition, the patient should also consult the other health experts such as the psychiatrist and dietician with regards to some psychological advices on long-term goals after the operation.

Generally, patients who have undergone weight loss surgery are said to be successful if they were able to lose 50% or more of their extra body weight and will be able to maintain that condition for the next five years or so. However, the results of the operation may still vary depending on the clinical information of the patient and the skills of the bariatric surgeon.

Normally, the patient will be able to lose at least 30% to a maximum of 50% during the first six months after surgery; and within the year after the operation, the patient has the potential of losing weight up to a maximum of 77%.

Best of all, people who were able to lose weight through surgical operations can actually maintain a continuous weight loss of up to 50% to 60% in the next 10 to 14 years after surgery.

Factors to Consider

As with the other weight loss management programs, there are many factors to consider before the patient should decide to undergo weight loss surgery.

Consequently, the actual weight that will be lost is reliant on the weight before surgery, surgical procedure, patient's age, capability to exercise, total health condition of the patient, dogged determination to maintain the necessary follow-up nurture, and the enthusiasm to succeed with the help of their family, friends, and their colleagues.

If you have just put on a few extra pounds and want to avoid gaining more, these weight loss surgeries for better health may seem convincing. But, in addition to being convinced, you may also have to take some action to ensure that your weight does not creep upward.

Therefore, it can be concluded that losing weight is not just a question of deciding to be strong-willed and determined or upbeat and positive. Lifestyle changes are where it is at for long-term success with your weight especially after weight loss surgery.

Tablets to Help in Weight Loss

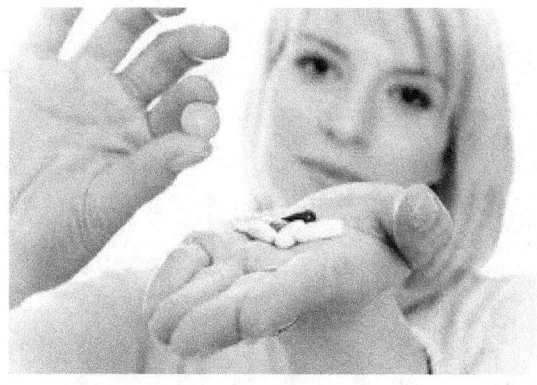

Recent studies have shown that more people are getting
overweight every year. This happens not only to adults
but even to kids who have just started in school.

There are many factors that have contributed to this such
as the rise in the number of fast foods joints that contain
a lot of saturated fat in the meals, the use of refined

sugar in sodas and other processed foods, eating food with less fiber, genetics, overeating and as people age slow metabolism.

Since losing weight takes time and most people can't wait to get rid of it, these people have decided to take the fastest way out which is through the use of weight loss tablets.

In the 1950's until the late 90's, doctors prescribed drugs for weight loss. The drug works by increasing the serotonin levels in the brain that makes the brain believe that the stomach is already full and thus, increases the person's metabolic rate.

It was only after scientists discovered that these drugs had side effects and were related to cause heart valve disease that these were taken off the shelves.

Later on, modifications have been made and new drugs were developed and prescribed by doctors and many of which are still waiting for FDA approval.

The idea that a simple drug can change everything without the need to change ones diet or sacrificing anything is very tempting since people have seen friends and family members use it and have shown tremendous improvement.

This has made a lot of people spend millions of dollars every year to also experience this miracle and has given drug companies a lot of money making the drug and selling it.

Diet pills can be purchased either over-the-counter or prescribed by a doctor. Even with the advances in medical technology, these drugs still pose a health risk to the public. Problems in patients can be unpleasant such as diarrhea and vomiting, harmful such as tightness in the chest and in the urinary tract and fatal such as a heart attack or a stroke.

An overdose in using weight loss tablets can cause tremors, confusion, hallucinations, shallow breathing, renal failure, heart attack and convulsions.

The side effects vary depending on the lifestyle and health of the person and can be minimized as long as one consults the doctor and follows the prescribed dosage when using it.

Should one decide to stop using the drugs, studies have shown that a person will experience withdrawal symptoms and side effects. These include noticeable mood swings, hyper-activity, and pain in the stomach, insomnia and nightmares, severe irritability, extreme fatigue, depression, nausea, vomiting and trembling.

A lot of clinical tests will show that the taking this weight loss tablets really work. But this can only work if it is done with a low calorie diet and an exercise plan.

A person can jog every morning or sign up and workout in a gym. Just like taking any medicine, one should first consult the doctor before undergoing any form of exercise.

The best exercise plan should have cardiovascular and weight training exercises. This helps burn calories and increase the muscle to fat ratio that will increase ones metabolism and lose weight.

It is up to the person already to stick to the program to see that it works.

Pointers on Losing Weight Safely

People, who want to lose weight commonly, and first of all, think about reducing the amount of food they eat.

This may be quite a solution but not exactly the best there is. In fact, depending on the amount you reduce in your food intake, it may even be dangerous to one's health.

So how does one lose weight effectively and safely? Here are some points one should consider when trying to lose weight:

Beware of the Crash Diets

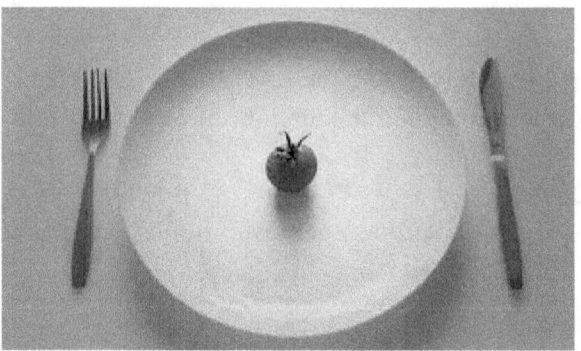

Most people think that trimming down the calories can alone shed off their unwanted excess. Probably this is because of the fad there is in advertising about low-calorie food products and beverages.

What people don't know is that this could be dangerous because when they decrease their calorie intake way to below the required levels, the body begins to digest the fats. Sounds good but it doesn't actually. Burning fat requires a lot of energy. Since there is not much energy in the body to facilitate metabolism of fat, it will run at a very slow pace resulting to fatigue, illness and weak immune system.

Low-calorie diet is also compensated for by the body by burning muscle. People on this type of diet who revert back to their old eating habits end up gaining back some; if not all the weight they have shed off.

This would consist mainly of fats. And since fats have more volume per mass than muscle, they end up having the same weight as before but more bulky.

In losing weight, one should keep in mind that they should lose excess body fats only.

However, one can try out eating small meals at more frequent intervals. This way the body will not think that it is being starved and will not store food as fat.

Eat Properly

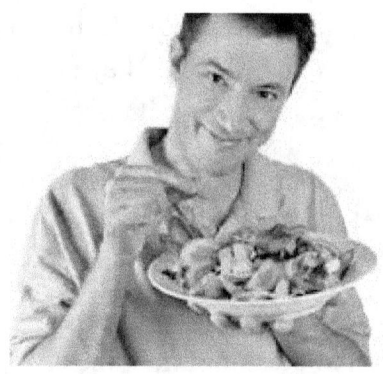

One may have considered junking the crash diet option but he should also not forget to watch what he is eating.

Variety must always be considered so that one may be able to get the necessary nutrients from his diet.

It is also healthier to eat foods which are roasted, steamed or broiled rather than fried. It is also important to include a lot of fiber in the diet. Frequent rehydration is also necessary.

Pump Up lean Muscle Mass

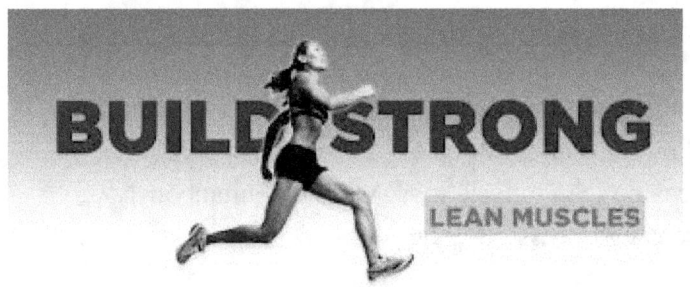

Muscles burn calories when they work; they even do so at rest. Unlike fats which just lie around, bulge around the pants and dangle beneath the sleeves, muscles burn calories all-day round.

With this fact, one can start weight loss by increasing muscle mass. The more muscles, the less fat will be left. This is attainable starting with working out with resistance exercises.

Engaging in Aerobics

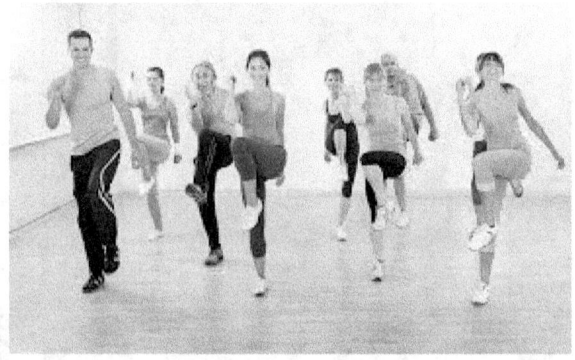

Aerobics are not only good for the heart by increasing cardio-vascular endurance. Aerobics also help in increasing lean muscle mass while simultaneously decreasing excess body fat.

Aside from these, aerobics make the metabolic process more efficient and its rate high, even after a long while. Imagine burning fat efficiently while driving along the freeway or even while watching television.

Extra "Push"

Some people believe that smoking and caffeine can actually help in losing weight. This can perhaps be true; however, they do the body more harm than good because of their side-effects.

For that extra "push", one can try out taking food supplements. After all, 95% of these products out in the market actually do well.

On Taking Diet Pills

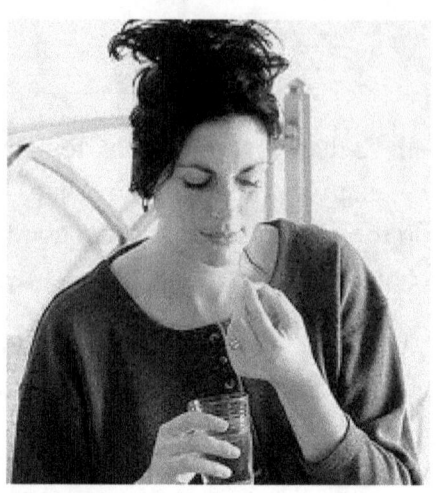

Over-the-counter diet pills affect the amount of weight one loses as well as how long one keeps that amount of weight off.

However, one must be wary of the side-effects of these diet pills. As such, one must faithfully follow the instructions provided for in the packaging.

It is also prudent to consult the physician anyway before trying out these drugs and also to find out which type would be best for the individual.

Losing weight does not have to mean sacrifice and suffering. It actually means opening up to a more full and healthy life where one may not have to feel bad about himself having to look the way he does or not being able to do what he wants to do.

Losing weight might entail a little adjustment plus the discomforts, but as the old saying goes, "no pain, no gain." Besides fat, what has one got to lose anyway?

Why Losing Weight is good

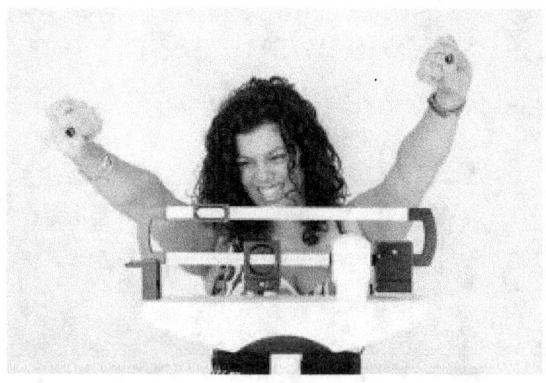

There is a great benefit acquired from losing weight. Though losing weight is not easy, the long term effects brought by it would probably be of help to anyone considering shedding those unwanted and unhealthy pounds.

The following are a few of the remarkable advantages from losing that excess weight.

Weight loss prevents high blood pressure, heart disease and stroke

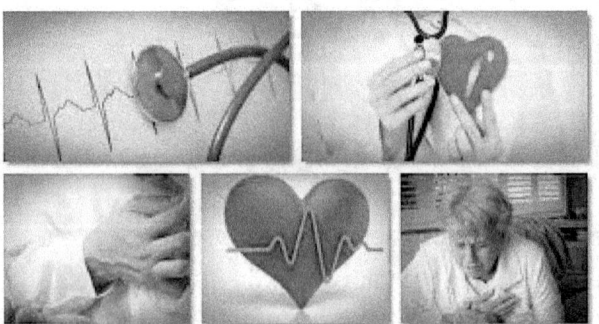

That is a three in one benefit from losing weight. It is a fact that heart disease and stroke are one of the primary reasons for disability and death in both men and women in the US.

People who are overweight have a higher risk to have high levels of cholesterol in their blood stream as well as triglycerides (also known as blood fat).

Angina, one type of heart disease, could cause chest pains as well as a decrease in the oxygen pumped to the heart.

Sudden death also occurs from heart disease and stroke, and usually this strikes with very little warning, signs and   symptoms.

It is a fact that by decreasing your weight by a mere five to ten percent, this could positively decrease the chances of you having or developing heart disease or a stroke.

Plus, how your heart functions would also improve as well as your blood pressure, cholesterol and triglyceride count will decrease.

Weight loss prevents type 2 diabetes

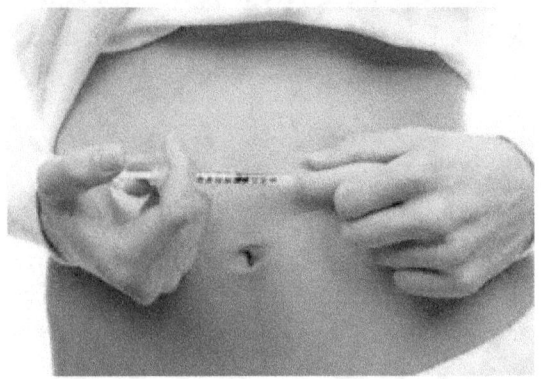

Diabetes puts in jeopardy one's life as well as how one leads his or her life because of the complications that result from having it.

Both types of diabetes, type one and type two are linked with being overweight.

To those who already have diabetes, regular exercise and losing weight could help in controlling your blood sugar levels as well as the medication you may be currently taking.

Increase your physical activity. You could simply walk, jog or dance. It helps get those blood streams moving as well as loses those unnecessary pounds.

Weight loss helps reduce your risk for cancer

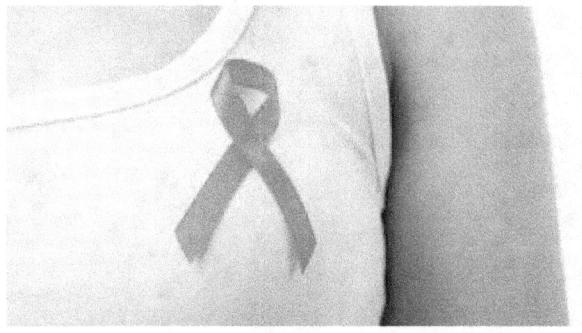

Being overweight is linked with a number of kinds of cancer. Especially for women, the common types of cancer that is associated with being overweight include cancer of the uterus, gallbladder, ovary, breast, and colon.

This is not meant to scare you; this is only to keep you informed. Men are at risk too from developing cancer if they are overweight.

These include cancer of the colon, prostate and rectum. Extra weight, a diet high in fat and cholesterol should as much as possible be avoided.

Weight loss reduces sleep apnea

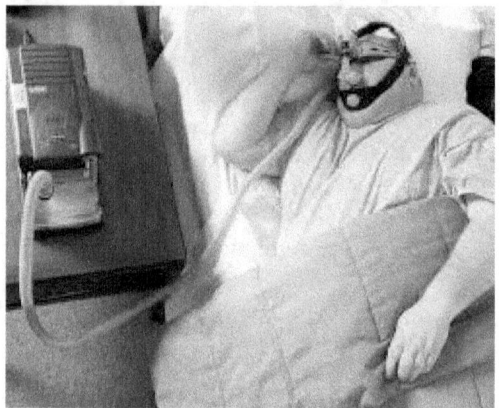

Or it could eliminate it all together. Sleep apnea is a condition wherein one could temporarily stop breathing for a brief period and then would continue to snore heavily.

Sleep apnea could cause drowsiness or sleepiness during the day and – because of being overweight – could result in heart failure. Shedding those excess pounds could help in eliminating this problem.

Weight loss reduces the pain of osteoarthritis

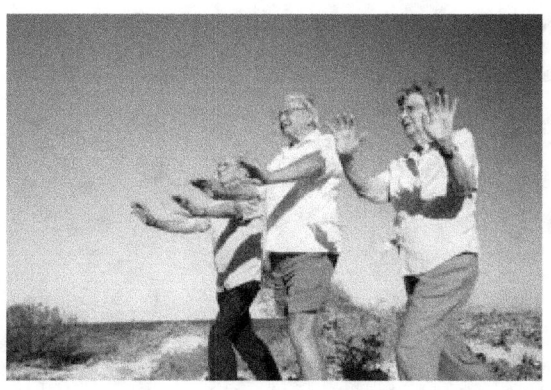

When one weighs heavily, the joints of his or her knees, hips and lower back would have to exert double – if not triple – effort to carry him or her throughout his / her waking, walking and moving life. This could cause tension and stress on these joints.

Weight loss decreases the load these joints carry thus decreasing – if not eliminating – the pain of one who has osteoarthritis.

"What there is to Know about Diet Pills?"

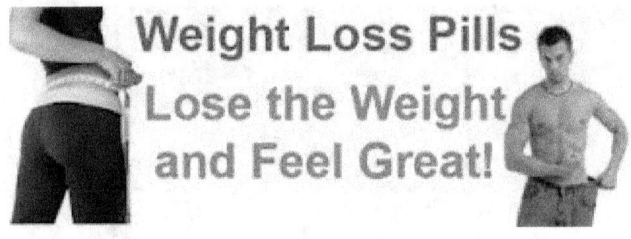

According to manufacturers, diet pills use natural ingredients capable of prolonging life and containing alcohol used in medication or flavoring.

One thing's for sure, never take diet pills as substitute for cutting calories without the doctor's recommendation. There are simple but important steps to be followed when taking diet pills:

1. Never crush diet pills to mix in drinks or soups. Take it whole with a full glass of water.

2. Diet pills cause a person to urinate more frequently due to its diuretic effect. This could lead to dehydration, thus, causing complications. As a pre-caution, it is best to drink eight glasses of water every day while on diet pills.

3. Take only the recommended dosage. Taking more than required will not help you lose weight but increase the risk of side effects.

4. Heartbeat should be less than 86 beats per minute. Stop taking the pills if it reaches 90 or higher that is why regular checking of pulse is a must.

5. Always follow the instructions set by the dietician and/or doctor and not only rely on what's enclosed in the box. Also diet pills will only work as expected if diet plan is being followed.

6. After three months, stop taking the diet pills. Common diet phenylpropanolamine is safe to use only up to sixteen weeks. Other studies show that it can cause health problems if taken under one month.

There are two kinds of diet pills; one is the prescription only diet pills and the over-the-counter diet pills.

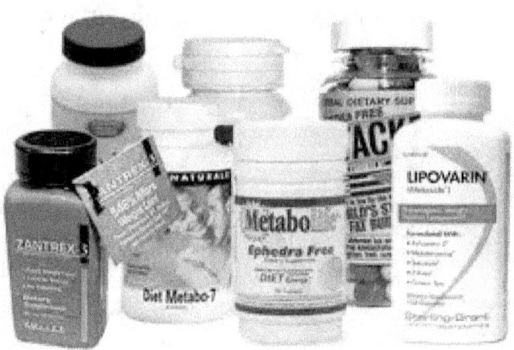

Prescription Diet Pills - are drugs regulated by the Food and Drug Administration agency which side effects are monitored, maybe advertised and prescribed under certain dosages.

The most popular of these is Xenical, which is licensed for long-term use. However, this too has its own side effects, diarrhea, oily and unexpected fecal discharges are just some. Therefore, users are advised to take a low fat diet plan.

While Over-the-Counter Diet Pills are categorized as food substitute and are unregulated. Beware that these diet pills are not Federal authorities tested and may cause serious side effects up to and including death.

Aside from a dietician, local pharmacists can also help in determining the pills that are safe and not for each person's case. Just be extra careful about the so-called "natural" or "organic" ingredients. Not everything that comes from a natural source is safe. One example is Ma Huang, which is a botanical source of ephedrine known as a stimulant and being studied for potential side effects.

Those who have or have a family history of prostate problems, thyroid disease, mental illness, high blood pressure, and heart problems should avoid taking diet supplements.

The same applies to those who've had seizures or strokes. If someone is taking cold medicines, especially those with decongestants, diet pills should not be taken.

Whether it is a prescription or an over-the-counter diet pill, the dangers are unvarying with other similar drug which control the brain to reduce appetite and includes chest pains, hair fall, fever, depression, and even impotence.

And as a general rule, don't ever try to take diet drugs if pregnancy is suspected. Persons that are allergic to sulfites and tartrazine should also avoid taking diet pills.

And those who are under 18 years or over 60 years of age should consult their doctor first prior to taking any dietary drugs, especially if they rely on over-the-counter stimulants used as a replacement for increase exercise.

"Nutrition Notes on Weight Loss Supplements"

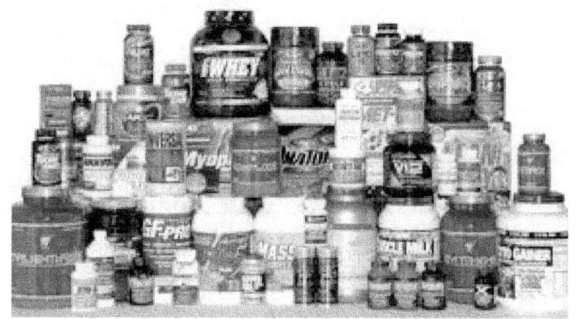

More and more spend hundred and even thousands of dollars yearly on weight loss supplements in the hope of speeding up their metabolism.

The main desire is to be attractive and accepted but it is becoming a more difficult goal to achieve.

The fitness industry is booming but still a lot of people are unable to cut those fats in spite of all the exercise and diet efforts.

In America, more than sixty per cent of adults are overweight and thirty per cent are considered obese.

This is because: one, a lot of weight loss products promises unrealistic goals; two, dietary supplement manufacturers rely on the overweight person's failure to survive; and three, the information about the supplements in the market are just written by themselves just to make a sell.

Although the Food and Drug Administration has successfully banned illegal marketers, some products are still available.

Consumers can be deceived of the labels which claims caffeine or ephedra fee not knowing that these supplements composes of other ingredients that may pose the same health risks.

These include heart and digestive problems, headaches, insomnia, and even psychological side effects.

Other supplement manufacturers say that their products contains EGCG which is a phytochemical ingredient found in green tea.

This so-called component claims to speed up metabolism but in reality poses to reduce the risk of cancer.

Some studies denote that it could slightly increase the potential to burn calories and now can be found in many weight loss supplements.

It has good points on the other hand since the body might conform to EGCG after a period of time.

Even the weight loss benefit could sum up to 60 to 70 calories a day. This helps prevent excessive weight gain.

A few other significant effects of weight loss supplements is that it may contain ingredients that makers claim will prevent the absorption of carbohydrates.

One good example is Chitosan, which appears most promising, which in fact shows no positive result in fat absorption.

It could even take up to seven months for men to lose just a pound of body fat and for women; there is no fat loss at all.

Thyroid supplements act as thyroid replacements help regulate and optimize the thyroid at a higher level.

This they say makes the body feel like a couch potato and won't perform the job it has to.

Since the number one reason why people eat is because they feel hungry, there is another type of ingredient that manufacturers made which increases the feeling of being full and decreases appetite, Guar Gum. However, recent studies show that it has no meaningful benefit at all to weight loss.

It is ironic that manufacturers mix Phylum that has the reputation of reducing eating and aiding weight loss for initial studies so far does not support this claim although it helps control blood cholesterol and sugar.

One of the latest innovations in the fat loss industry is by way of skin absorption. There's a Cutting Gel, which is an epidural product by far the best selling in fat loss creams technology.

Rub it where you want the fats cut. For now, it will seem safer to advise the age old remedies to excessive weight gain and that is to invest in walking shoes instead of diet supplements, go to the park and do brisk some walking, go to the gym, and have a well-balanced diet instead.